HOW THE APA NORMALIZED HOMOSEXUALITY

J.P. Sloane, M.A., Ph.D.

AvingtonHouse Publishing

HOW THE APA NORMALIZED HOMOSEXUALITY

By J.P. Sloane, Ph.D.

ISBN: 979-8-9961594-3-7
AvingtonHouse Publishing, Dallas

In regard to this issue, we do not wish to attack any person for their sexuality, nor justify their choices. We intend to report on the various sources and the consequences inferred when dealing with this subject from historical, scientific, religious, and political perspectives.

A note on sources used. Until recently, we preferred to use most of our documentation from tangible sources such as books, magazines, and newspapers, rather than digital sources. The Internet is rife with questionable documentation because revisionists can delete the original source or replace it with their own agenda. *Wikipedia* has been the subject of that and, consequently, is somewhat suspect as a source, so we double-check their sources on the topics we research with them to make sure they are legitimate. That said, most credible sources today have moved online because of cost and distribution efficiency, which also makes them easier for readers to access and verify. One example is The Encyclopædia Britannica, which has been published exclusively online since 2016. When using the Internet as a source, we make every effort to ensure that sources are verifiable, respected, and mainstream, such as the highly esteemed Encyclopædia Britannica.

WHY A BOOK LIKE THIS NOW?

We are addressing the subject of how homosexuality became normalized in response to the many people who are disturbed by what they see as a great destructive uproar and indecency in our society, including naked men parading in public, and boys and men showering alongside girls and women. The legalization of same-sex marriage has promoted the proliferation of rainbow flags at protests and on government buildings, not to mention transsexuals exposing themselves on the lawn of the Biden White House. This book is in response to their requests for an understanding of what is happening in today's society and how it's affecting all of us. In doing so, we examine how medical professionals, rather than relying on empirical science, choose to approach a mental disorder through a more democratic process. By allowing emotions and intimidation, among some in the community of psychiatrists and psychologists, these medical professionals elected to avoid science in reclassifying what was once considered a mental disorder or sickness as now being perfectly normal by those members of the American Psychiatric Association (APA).

In this book, we will explore some of the disturbing background that led to the removal of that condition from the APA's

Diagnostic and Statistical Manual of Mental Disorders.

In this instance, the former disorder was homosexuality, but the same means of normalization could just as easily be applied to PTSD (Post-Traumatic Stress Disorder), ADHD (Attention-Deficit/Hyperactivity Disorder), and various other ailments listed in the Diagnostic and Statistical Manual of Mental Disorders. Therefore, rest assured that in dealing with the subject of normalizing homosexuality, we will not be singling them out for moral or political reasons, but to respond to those who are confused about how the new WOKE political agenda governing our healthcare systems is managed and to address those concerns.

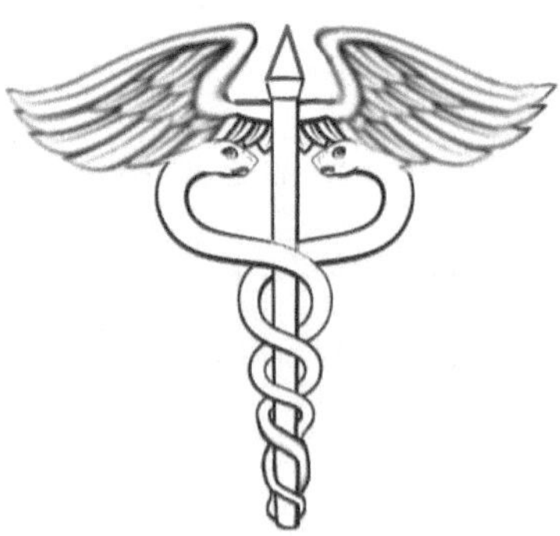

Table of Contents

INTRODUCTION

This book is an exposé for those curious about what motivated the doctors of the American Psychiatric Association to normalize homosexuality in its official publication, the *Diagnostic and Statistical Manual of Mental Disorders*, thereby creating normalcy out of something that obviously does not function in the way and for the purpose for which the plumbing was intended. So, we must ask, was it empirical science (experimental observation and verification through data collection and evaluation) or something else that caused the change? While we don't want to be overly technical or contentious, we have chosen to publish this condensed book to provide an overview of how what was once considered an abnormal sexual relation is now understood as normal and to help inform readers about the facts surrounding it. For the reason that religion has played a large part throughout history regarding sex, it is something we cannot avoid, although we make every effort not to be preachy and to stay as neutral as possible.

In this publication, we will explore for those who are curious about how a medical condition can be neutralized through a social procedure known as *demedicalization*, which is the process by which a condition, behavior, or natural life process loses its definition as a medical "disease" or pathology and is instead recategorized as a normal variation of life or a social issue.[1] In this case, by avoiding science, and for those of you who are concerned about how the status of normalization was accomplished.

Since we are dealing with a specific anomaly, we must provide all the relevant history and ramifications surrounding it. While this can be very tedious and complex, this volume is not intended as an exhaustive study of homosexual behavior and how it became normalized. Rather, it is an overview of the key factors by which homosexuality was made an acceptable indulgence. Many excellent books—some of which we have

---

[1]Joel T. Braslow and Luke Messac, "Medicalization and Demedicalization — A Gravely Disabled Homeless Man with Psychiatric Illness," ed. Scott D. Stonington et al., *New England Journal of Medicine* 379, no. 20 (November 15, 2018): 1885–88, https://doi.org/10.1056/nejmp1811623.

drawn from and listed in the footnotes—provide far greater detail and documentation for readers who wish to explore this topic further.

To be sure, some of the chapters, although short, can also be a little technical. One example: because sexuality includes both plants and animals, we will explore and deal with the beginning of life from the Darwinian secular theory,[2] which is taught in schools, although as a Christian, I find that Creation Science provides many challenges to Darwin's theory that, after 150 years, has never been proven and is still just a theory.[3] Nevertheless, because we are addressing a general audience, both secular and religious, we will adopt a neutral perspective.

On the subject of religion, we must acknowledge that religions have historically played a major role in sex,[4] and therefore we must unavoidably address it when dealing with this topic.[5] However, our research will primarily focus on the secular

---

[2] Charles Darwin. *On THE ORIGIN OF SPECIES or PREVISION OF FAVORED RACES IN THE STRUGGLE FOR LIFE* . (London, John Murray Publisher, 1859)

[3] Michael J. Behe. *DARWIN'S BLACK BOX: THE BIOCHEMICAL CHALLENGE TO* EVOLUTION (New York, A TOUCHSTONE BOOK PUBLISHED BY SIMON & SCHUSTER, 6th Edition, 2003).

[4] Carolyn Sprague, MA, review of *Religion and Sexuality | EBSCO*, EBSCO Information Services, Inc. | www.ebsco.com, 2023,

[5] Federico Lega. *Elgar Encyclopedia of Healthcare Management*. (Cheltenham, UK: Edward Elgar Publishing, 2023).

aspects of the gay or homosexual lifestyles. That being said, we must also address the various aspects of sex throughout the ages, as sexual conduct has historically been affected by it. Be assured that while we will not dwell on religious issues, some must be addressed to bring historical accuracy and balance to the topic of sex and its practices.

Before we begin, I should share—for the sake of background—that I was born into an entertainment family in Hollywood, California, and was privileged to start in show business at a very early age, appearing on radio, television, and in motion pictures, as well as being one of the youngest persons ever to be under contract with Universal Studios.[6] By the time I was nine years old, I had appeared on the covers of five magazines distributed throughout the Free World. Each magazine sold over one million copies. In my late teens, I embarked on a career as a recording artist. I am not revealing this to brag about myself, but to show how I was immersed in the entertainment industry from an early age. In that industry, there are numerous homosexuals, and I knew and worked with many of them. Personally, we do not care about their private lives, as it is none of our business, and our private life is also none of theirs. I have never had a problem knowing or working

---

[6] J.P. Sloane-Biography-IMDB (Internet Movie Data Base).

with "Gay" people or anyone else; all that matters to me is that you are pleasant to work with and are accomplished and professional in the delivery of your theatrical talent(s).

In the same way that my private life is my business and your private life is your business, I have no reason to tell you how you should live your life unless, of course, you ask my advice (I have an earned Master's Degree in Counseling).

While I personally try to live my life according to the Judeo-Christian Bible, to be honest, I do not always agree with God, but ultimately, I know who is right, and to my chagrin, it is not me!

Having shared that, we will now embark on the scandal surrounding the history of how homosexuality came to be normalized by the American Psychiatric Association, the method by which it was removed from the APA's Diagnostic and Statistical Manual of Mental Disorders, and the repercussions that followed.

CHAPTER ONE

STARTING AT THE DARWINIAN BEGINNING

Because we are dealing with the makeup and reproduction of all life forms, concluding with human sexuality, it becomes necessary to begin at the beginning by visiting the secular viewpoint of how life started. Due to the tedious nature of this subject, we will provide only an overview of the main technical points, keeping it to a few pages.

It should not be surprising that currently, there are many areas of controversy surrounding human sexuality and the so-called animal nature of man in today's society. First, the premise rests on accepting, as a fact, the evolutionist view (which is still only a theory) that all life (plants and animals) evolved from a simple-celled, ancient anaerobic bacterium that did not require oxygen.[7] This first life form supposedly arose after eons of inanimate molecules in a primordial soup repeatedly bumped into each other aimlessly like balls on a pool table —until a group of them, uncannily, made simultaneous contact at just the right angles and points in time. We are told that this assembly of coincidental, simultaneous events allowed an energetic, self-directing life force to be infused into the new entity's molecular conglomeration, culminating in the original parental form of all living things on our planet. Of course, what this newly created biological life form is and where the energizing life force itself came from are inexplicable outside of a creator. Given the odds of more than one original life form being spontaneously created, it would seem more likely that the first crude life form would have been algae. Nevertheless, because Earth's atmosphere had very little oxygen, the first life form would need to breathe something other than oxygen, ruling out algae. We must also consider what it ate and how it reproduced; probably, it used cell division. Perhaps, although highly unlikely and against all odds, there may have been many

---

[7] Madeline C. Weiss et al., "The Physiology and Habitat of the Last Universal Common Ancestor," *Nature Microbiology* 1, no. 9 (July 25, 2016), https://doi.org/10.1038/nmicrobiol.2016.116.

anaerobic bacteria that were miraculously formed at the same time?[8] Your guess is as good as any.

THE VARIOUS MEANS OF REPRODUCTION, INCLUDING SEX

For life to reproduce itself, two primary forms of reproduction are required. The anaerobic bacterium (Darwin's first simple cell life form) was asexual (i.e., sexually neutral, or genderless) because, according to Darwin, it was most likely that only one creation event occurred. Consider the challenge for this proto, or first life form, to reproduce itself without another of its kind—like heterosexual creatures must do—if later life forms were to evolve from it. This required a reproduction process known as binary fission, which allows reproduction when the single parent cell divides into two daughter cells, thereby producing replicas of the original anaerobic bacterium.

Asexual reproduction[9] is important because, as stated above, it allows offspring to be produced from a single parent and allows them to inherit the parent's genes. This type of reproduction

---

[8] Editors of Science News Today. (2025). New Study Reveals Life on Earth May Be Far More Unlikely Than We Ever Imagined. In *Science News Today*. https://www.sciencenewstoday.org/new-study-reveals-life-on-earth-may-be-far-more-unlikely-than-we-ever-imagined

[9] University of Utah, "Sexual vs. Asexual Reproduction," Utah.edu, 2016, https://learn.genetics.utah.edu/content/basics/reproduction/.

rarely involves meiosis (the process by which a cell divides twice, forming four cells each with half the genetic information), ploidy (the number of complete sets of chromosomes in a cell), or fertilization (the combination of a paternal sperm nucleus combining with a maternal egg nucleus forming an embryo).

Hermaphrodites are life forms that have both male and female reproductive organs, including snails, some fish, and most plants. Occasionally, but very rarely, a human can be born with a condition classified as hermaphroditism, which is not to be confused with being a transvestite. Unlike the animal hermaphrodites, the human hermaphrodites cannot engage in sexual activity by themselves. This is one of the rarest forms of disorders of sexual differentiation (DSD) in humans, representing only 5% of all human births.[10] Animal hermaphrodites can engage in sexual activity with another hermaphrodite, using both sexual organs simultaneously.[11]

---

[10] Muhammad Zafar Iqbal et al., "True Hermaphrodite: A Case Report," *APSP Journal of Case Reports* 2, no. 2 (July 30, 2011): 16, https://pmc.ncbi.nlm.nih.gov/articles/pmc3418019/.

[11] Britannica Editors, "Hermaphroditism | Definition, Types, & Effects," Encyclopedia Britannica, July 20, 1998, https://www.britannica.com/science/hermaphroditism.

Another means of reproduction is heterosexual reproduction, which requires a male and a female with a highly developed means of delivering sperm to the ovum, resulting in the fertilization of an egg contained in the female of the species. Humans reproduce their kind in this manner. However, we know that—aside from the virgin birth of Jesus—certain heterosexual reptiles and amphibians that reproduce through the interaction of the male and female of the species are able, albeit rarely, to reproduce in a manner not completely understood without male impregnation. This phenomenon is called parthenogenesis.[12]

However, when dealing with human sexuality, reproduction through sexual intercourse is the primary biological means by which humans and other highly advanced organisms conceive and give birth to children. This process requires genetic material from both parents, resulting in the fusion of specific reproductive cells, known as gametes, to generate genetically distinct offspring.

As for exceptions, we have the famous John B. Calhoun behavioral sink experiments conducted on rodent populations,

---

[12]R. A. Beatty, *Parthenogenesis and Polyploidy in Mammalian Development (Cambridge Monographs in Experimental Biology),* First edition, (Cambridge: Cambridge University Press, 1957).

which showed that under extreme overpopulation and crowding, the rats' social structures completely broke down, resulting in a variety of abnormal behaviors, including same-sex mounting and a loss of regular mating.[13]

Therefore, aside from believing that a human male or female was subjected to the wrong body at birth, which requires the belief in a spiritual world—a dimension which usually contains a god whose nature, in the Judeo-Christian sense, could not make such a mistake—and considering the fact that most religions condemn homosexuality, we must look for other possibilities to normalize homosexual behavior in humans.

---

[13] Edmund Ramsden and Jon Adams, "Escaping the Laboratory: The Rodent Experiment of John B. Calhoun and Their Cultural Influence," *Journal of Social History* 42, no. 3 (2026): 761–97,

CHAPTER TWO

WHAT CHANGED HOMOSEXUALITY FROM ABNORMAL TO NORMAL?

For millennia, it was thought that a biological entity that is heterosexual in design yet has no desire to reproduce through its biological coupling mechanism was considered queer or perverted because it departed from its normal reproductive function. Revisiting heterosexuality for a moment and allowing that the process of giving birth is very painful, an overriding desire must be initiated in females that causes them to desire intimacy with a man, an intimacy which inevitably leads to a pregnancy and the resulting birthing process. However, reproduction in any species, from the lowly anaerobic bacterium to human beings, is for the continuation of the species. Yet now, where humans are concerned, it has been redirected to allow not just a man and a woman, but a man and a man or a woman and a woman as well! What caused this reclassification of homosexuality, equating it to that of the natural heterosexual predisposition and nature's physical design for the male/female sexual encounter—along with its intended result for the continuation of the human species—as being equally acceptable and normal? What caused the normalization of homosexual behavior being taught in our classrooms to heterosexual children, and promoting the alternative possibility that some boys really were girls in a boy's body, as well as the same thing for girls and suggesting that it was perfectly normal for boys to want to be with boys and girls with girls—which with prepubescent children is predictably normal—but now they are exposed to accepting their dislike of the icky other sex and their like for kids of their own sex in a more physical way (male on male, female on female)? How and why is homosexual desirability now promoted as an accepted and normal alternative behavior being taught to pre-adolescent kids? Was it due to strenuous scientific laboratory observations and exhaustive, unflawed empirical testing?

Consider Ronald Bayer, Ph.D., a professor at the Center for the History and Ethics of Public Health at the Mailman School of

Public Health, Columbia University,[14] where he has taught for many years and has been involved with the homosexual community in a positive way regarding homosexuality. Dr. Bayer has shown insightfulness through his book regarding psychology and psychiatry's disciplines and the basis for the reversal of homosexuality as a psychiatric disorder and how it came to be normalized in his bestselling and highly recommended book, *Homosexuality and American Psychiatry: The Politics of Diagnosis*,[15]

---

[14]Ronald Bayer, Ph. D. Prior to Dr. Bayer having come to Columbia he was at the Hastings Center, a research institute devoted to the study of ethical issues in medicine and the life sciences. Bayer's research has examined ethical and policy issues in public health. His empirical work has focused especially on AIDS, tuberculosis, illicit drugs, and tobacco. His broader project is to develop an ethics of public health. He is an elected member of the IOM, on its Board on Health Promotion and Disease Prevention and has served on IOM committees dealing with the social impact of AIDS, tuberculosis elimination, vaccine safety, smallpox vaccination and the Ryan White Care Act. His articles on AIDS have appeared in the *New England Journal of medicine, The Journal of the American Medical Association, The Lancet, the American Journal of Public Health*, and *The Milbank Quarterly*. His books include *Homosexuality and American Psychiatry: The Politics of Diagnosis* (1981), *Private Acts, Social Consequences: AIDS and the Politics of Public Health* (1989); *AIDS in the Industrialized Democracies: Passions, Politics and Policies* (1991, edited with David Kirp); *Confronting Drug Policy: Illicit Drugs in a Free Society* (1993, edited with Gerald Oppenheimer); and *Blood Feuds: Blood, AIDS and the Politics of Medical Disaster* (1999, edited with Eric Feldman); *AIDS Doctors: Voices from the Epidemic,* (2000, written with Gerald Oppenheimer and Mortal Secrets: Truth and Lies in the Age of AIDS (2003, co-authored with Robert Klitzman). <http://www.columbia.edu/itc/hs/medical/bioethics/egir/cv/Bayer.pd> Accessed 1 April, 2013.

[15]Ronald Bayer, Ph.D., *Homosexuality and American Psychiatry: The Politics of Diagnosis* (Princeton: Princeton University Press, 1987)

In dealing with the issue of homosexuality, normal vs. abnormal, we will present several excellent examples that expose the flawed concepts concerning the so-called science of psychology and psychiatry and how these alleged medical disciplines fall short of actually qualifying as a science.

For most people, it is not surprising that homosexuality has been regarded for most of recorded history as a deviant (to turn away from) unnatural behavior. However, with the advent of the political and sexual revolution in the 1960s, the morals of the 1950s were summarily abandoned, and the expression, "If it feels good, DO IT!" became the cry of a lost generation. Now, over half a century later, those rebellious flower children of the 1960s social revolt have ascended to positions of power among today's movers and shakers. Tenured professors follow in Timothy Leary's[16] footsteps, using unorthodox methods and morals to mold children's minds from kindergarten through grad school. Thus, it was no surprise that along with the civil rights and women's rights movements, the homosexual

---

[16]Timothy Francis Leary (October 22, 1920--May 31, 1996) was an American psychologist and writer, known for his advocacy of psychedelic drugs.... During the 1960s and 1970s, he was arrested often enough to see the inside of 29 different prisons worldwide. President Richard Nixon once described Leary as "the most dangerous man in America". <http://en.wikipedia.org/wiki/Timothy_Leary> Accessed 1 April, 2013.

community would also begin to flex its muscles against society's norms, demanding not only acceptance but preference.

While conducting research on the Internet regarding the promotion of the LGBTQ agenda in children's programming, we came across this Google "AI" observation:

> Children's television programming has increasingly included LGBTQ+ characters and storylines to reflect diverse family structures and promote inclusivity. Networks and streaming platforms maintain that this representation aims to normalize different types of families and teach acceptance to young viewers.[17]

Predictably, this shift has sparked intense societal debate. Some advocacy groups, such as the Concerned Women for America, argue that shows on platforms like Netflix,[18] Disney,[19]

---

[17] Josie Powell, "16 Kids Shows with LGBTQIA+ Characters and Storylines," Care.com Resources, June 9, 2023, https://www.care.com/c/kids-shows-with-lgbtq-characters-and-storylines/.

[18] Samantha Kamman, "Netflix's Promotion of LGBT Themes, Sexual Preferences in Kids' Shows 'Pervasive': Report," Christianpost.com (The Christian Post, December 11, 2025), https://www.christianpost.com/news/netflixs-promotion-of-lgbt-themes-to-kids-pervasive-report.html.

[19] Akash Nikolas, "The Pro-Gay Message Hidden In Every Disney Film," The Atlantic (The Atlantic, April 23, 2014),

and PBS push adult topics, gender identity, and a "homosexual agenda"[20] onto young children without sufficient parental warning. In contrast, LGBTQ organizations like GLAAD[21] advocate for these storylines, arguing that they provide vital support and visibility for queer youth and help all children understand the diversity of their communities.

Agenda-Driven Lobby, Not Science, **Forced the Change**

The arrival of the 1970s brought a concentrated effort by the homosexual community to change homosexuality from being perceived as abnormal to normal. Their pressure began to be felt by the APA (American Psychiatric Association). Because of this book's chapter constraints, we will not delve in-depth into the highly complex and divergent twists and turns that led to the monumental certification process that allowed homosexuality to become regarded as perfectly normal behavior. Instead, we will touch on some of those events that

---

https://www.theatlantic.com/entertainment/archive/2014/04/its-not-just-frozen-disney-has-always-been-subtly-pro-gay/361060/.

[20] Andrea Morris, "Children's Show 'Odd Squad' Becomes Latest PBS Kids Show to Feature Same-Sex Marriage," CBN, July 17, 2022, https://cbn.com/news/us/childrens-show-odd-squad-becomes-latest-pbs-kids-show-feature-same-sex-marriage.

[21] Sarah Kate Ellis, AKA Sarahkateellis "Instagram," Instagram.com, 2026, https://www.instagram.com/p/duwfm0gdmor/.

led to the nomenclature (i.e., terminology, jargon, vocabulary) change regarding the normalization of homosexual behavior in the APA's official *Diagnostic and Statistical Manual of Psychiatric Disorders.*

The time is 1970; the place is San Francisco, California; the event is a meeting of the *American Psychiatric Association*. To San Francisco's homosexual community, this event was too good an opportunity to let pass unnoticed. It was not long before they quickly organized a protest voicing their outrage against the nomenclature of homosexuality as a mental illness in the APA's *Diagnostic and Statistical Manual of Psychiatric Disorders*. Lesbian and homosexual groups banded together in the first organized effort to disrupt and bring anarchy to the American Psychiatric Association convention. Outrageous behavior was the order of the day, with homosexual activists shouting violent verbal attacks, which spilled over to an APA committee meeting on "issues of sexuality."[22]

Because of the homosexual community's intimidating behavior, it was agreed by the APA that there could be a homosexual

---

[22]Reports appeared in the *Washington Post*, and the *San Francisco Chronicle*, May 15, 1970 editions, as well as the *Washington Star*, May 24, 1970.

presence at their next convention in Washington, D.C. That concession would allow the activists a forum to present their demands directly to the APA's leadership; "... it was clear that only the threat of disorder or even violence had been able to create the conditions out of which such a dialogue could occur. That lesson would not be forgotten."[23]

The leaders of the APA desired to avoid confrontation with homosexual activists at all costs. In May 1971, at the Washington, D.C. convention, it was even decided not to have a visible uniformed security presence, hoping to "ride out" any confrontation demonstration that was sure to occur. Homosexual activist Frank Kameny took a page from a Vietnam protester and stormed the prestigious APA's "Convocation of Fellows," shouting, "Psychiatry is the enemy incarnate. Psychiatry has waged a relentless war of extermination against us. You may take this as a declaration of war against you!"[24] Thus, it should be of no surprise that at that convention, homosexual activists gained entry and access to virtually every area they wanted to insert themselves by using forged credentials. Once they gained access to the exhibit area, they

---

[23]Ronald Bayer, Ph.D., *Homosexuality and American Psychiatry*, 104.

[24]*The Advocate*, (a homosexual and lesbian news magazine) May 26, 1971, 3.

"...came across a display marketing aversive conditioning techniques for the treatment of homosexuals," so they demanded that it be removed by threatening to tear down the exhibit if they didn't! The booth was removed.

Conversely, at the 1972 Dallas convention of the APA, there was a more subdued interaction by the homosexual activists "...since the Psychiatric Association had accommodated itself to the inevitability of homosexual pressure...."[25] The APA created a special panel to discuss homosexuality, consisting of a homosexual psychiatrist who concealed his identity behind the name of "Dr. Anonymous" and declared, "I am a homosexual. I am a psychiatrist."[26] This may have had the desired result of having the heterosexual members of the APA left wondering, "Who or how many anonymous homosexual psychiatrists there were?"[27]

Finally, at the 1973 convention, after many back-door discussions, confrontations, violent actions, and threats, it was

---

[25] Ibid., 107-108.

[26] Fryer, John Ercel. "Preserving American Freedom." *Robert Palmer Knight / Exhibits.hsp.org*, <http://digitalhistory.hsp.org/pafrm/person/robert-palmer-knight.> (Accessed 24, April 2022.) This site has many documents including "Dr. Henry Anonymous' " [John Fryer] handwritten notes used at the American Psychiatric Association 125th Annual Meeting

[27] Ibid.

decided that a vote should be taken. Regarding the events moving toward that climax, Dr. Bayer writes:

> In an effort to create a receptive climate for his presentation at the Nomenclature meeting, Silverstein enlisted a number of sympathetic psychiatrists and psychologists to address the committee with statements supporting the deletion of homosexuality from the Diagnostic and Statistical Manual. Seymour Halleck—a psychiatrist widely acknowledged as a critic of the abuse of psychiatric authority—wrote that scientific evidence was lacking to support the view that homosexuality was a developmental disorder and stated that homosexual behavior could best be considered a "common behavior[al] variant." (Dashes substituted for commas, ours)[28]

The fact that no scientific evidence supporting the claim that homosexuality is normal was presented by the homosexual lobby, the APA was nonetheless persuaded through intimidation to move quickly to delete homosexuality as a mental disorder from the *Diagnostic and Statistical Manual of Psychiatric Disorders.* In fact, "... the Nomenclature Committee had been so eager to bring the discussion of homosexuality to

---

[28] Ronald Bayer. *Homosexuality and American Psychiatry: The Politics of Diagnosis.* (Prinston: Prinston University Press, 1987), 117

a predetermined resolution that they had repeatedly violated accepted procedures for the consideration of such matters."[29] Usually, a special task force would have been empowered to investigate the matter under consideration and report its findings to the council. In doing so, the committee would usually defer to the task force's resulting conclusions. To override the task force's conclusions would be a dramatic departure from established precedent and "represent a violation of the principles of scientific authority." However, through pressure from many sources, a new precedent would be forthcoming.

> In an atmosphere charged with both anticipation and unflagging [tireless] militancy, there were demands for a 'gay presence' at the board's meeting. Threats of mobilizing a major picket of APA headquarters were made. (Bracketed clarification ours.)[30]

To calm things down and present a united front to defuse the predictable skepticism of removing homosexuality as a mental disorder from the *DSM-II* (*Diagnostic and Statistical Manual of Psychiatric Disorders*) and add credibility to what some in the

---

[29]Ibid., 132.
[30]Ibid., 134.

public community would see as a denial of reality, it was agreed to have a joint press conference of homosexual activists and leaders of the APA.

Nevertheless, Dr. McDevitt[31] saw it otherwise and disputed the encroaching redefinition of homosexuality, arguing that clinical observations reinforced the abnormality of homosexual attraction and that by revising the terminology, it had to be because of "political and philosophical grounds."[32]

To further influence the vote allowing the normalization of same-sex attractions, the homosexual lobby—composed overwhelmingly of homosexual psychiatrists—obtained a mailing list of APA members' names and addresses. It was also instrumental in financing the direct mailing cost, which ran about $2,500 in an unethical but successful attempt to sway the vote in their favor.[33] From the very beginning, scandal surrounded the entire process of normalizing homosexuality

---

[31] Legacy, "John McDevitt Obituary (2007) - New York, NY - New York Times," Legacy.com (Legacy, November 22, 2007), https://www.legacy.com/us/obituaries/nytimes/name/john-mcdevitt-obituary?id=33083155.

[32] Karla Jay and Allen Young (eds.). *Out of the Closets: Voices of Gay Liberation* (New York: Jove Books, 1972), 147. Under the heading *Surviving Psychotherapy,* citing Christopher Z. Hobson.

[33] Ronald Bayer. *Homosexuality and American Psychiatry:* 145.

through threats, intimidation, lobbying, and direct mailing scams, which raised many an eyebrow at the vote itself. When the vote to declare that homosexuality was not a disease or mental disorder finally arrived, it was passed under a cloud of those unethical procedures.

Dr. Socaride argued that important information had been withheld, resulting in a reversal of the vote's outcome, which made homosexuality normal. If that were not enough, Dr. Redlich's committee condemned using the referendum to affect the outcome of the homosexual agenda and the board of trustees' conduct in avoiding dealing with the scientific challenges.[34]

During the December 1974 meeting, the Board of Trustees agreed with Dr. Redlich's findings regarding unethical behavior surrounding the homosexual reclassification affair. In light of that finding, the board approved recommendations for public disclosure of all material intended to influence members of the Association.

> The trustees sidestepped, however, the difficult question of the appropriate role of referenda in

---

[34]Ibid., 153.

'scientific' and 'nonscientific' disputes. Having experienced the consequences of their action on homosexuality, they sought to avoid a potentially disruptive debate on this fundamental question, which touched on the scientific status of psychiatry.[35]

ANOTHER PROMINENT MEDICAL ASSOCIATION ADMITS THEY ALSO BYPASSED SCIENCE

As if that wasn't enough, The Federalist recently reported that the highly respected professional-medical organization, the *World Professional Association for Transgender Health* (WPATH):

> (WPATH) has been treated as incontestable expert guidance. Deep blue states like California have used WPATH standards to expand access to transgender interventions for children, and to force health insurance companies to cover sex-rejecting procedures. Believe in science!

[35] Ibid.,154.

But to their chagrin, WPATH had to admit before a court of law that all of its affirmation regarding transgender people was only a guess, and its guidance was only opinion![36]

> WPATH has conceded in court that its "Standards of Care" is merely an opinion. WPATH says it represents one side of an unsettled scientific debate marked by uncertainty — and physicians & orgs that rely on WPATH as the standard of care must bear "independent responsibility."[37]

When you ignore science, even for the best of intentions, it can come back to bite you!

[36] Chris Bray "Suddenly The Radical Pro-Trans Medical Organization WPATH Tells A Court That It's Just Guessing." *The Federalist*, A DIVISON OF FDRLST MEDIA, 12 Aug. 2026, thefederalist.com/2026/08/12/suddenly-the-radical-pro-trans-medical-organization-wpath-tells-a-court-that-its-just-guessing/.

[37] Ibid.

CHAPTER THREE

IN DEFENSE OF HOMOSEXUALITY AND ITS UNINTENDED CONSEQUENCES

Consider if you were to visit the Psychology Department at a university today and inquire about the normality of homosexuality, you would be assured that homosexuality is a perfectly acceptable, normal behavior. You would also find similar information as that found on the Wikipedia website:

> Since the 1970s, the consensus of the behavioral and social sciences and the health and mental health professions globally is that homosexuality is a normal variation of human sexual orientation, while there remain those who maintain that it is a disorder. In 1973, the *American Psychiatric Association* declassified homosexuality as a mental disorder. The *American Psychological Association Council of Representatives* followed in 1975. After that,

> other major mental health organizations followed, and it was finally declassified by the World Health Organization in 1990. Consequently, while some still believe homosexuality is a mental disorder, the current research and clinical literature demonstrate that same-sex sexual and romantic attractions, feelings, and behaviors are normal and positive variations of human sexuality, reflecting the official positions of the *American Psychiatric Association and the American Psychological Association*.[38]

This type of rhetoric is now the consensus across the behavioral and social sciences, as well as the health and mental health professions, globally. Today—based solely on a vote which is hardly a scientific approach—homosexuality is now accepted as a perfectly normal variation of human sexual orientation. A college student might very well be told by the Psychology Department that some misguided religious bigots still hold on to biblical myths about an angry God who hates those who "share alternative forms of affection and love." The student would be cautioned that modern individuals, when dealing with the phenomenon of same-sex attractions in homosexual couples, would be wise not to rely on the

---

[38]Homosexuality and psychology <http://en.wikipedia.org/wiki/Homosexuality_and_psychology> Accessed 29 March, 2013.

Judeo-Christian perspective or the sexual views of Muslims or any other religion for that matter.

Surprisingly, we would agree with the psychology professor that one does not need to rely on religion regarding homosexuality because same-sex attraction transcends both religion and psychology which can be addressed outside of both those disciplines. To demonstrate this concept, let us now consider a young college graduate whose family, and he, are ranchers—after being taught that homosexuality is entirely normal—he is troubled by an investment he made concerning two prize bulls that he bought for breeding. He kept them together in an exclusive private pen, hoping to produce even more prize bulls. Nevertheless, because nothing has come of this, he decides to double-check what he was taught in college by the psychology professor. He returns to the University seeking reconfirmation that what he is trying to do is perfectly normal. He asks the professor of counseling whether he understood correctly, when he was a student, that males having sex with other males is an acceptable, normal behavior. The professor assures him that it is and that even animals do it. Then, as he leaves the Psychology Department, he spots the Biology Department across the hall and decides he should also seek advice from that department about what he is doing wrong with his two bulls, because the Biology Department deals with animals and may have ideas that could help him. So, he inquires of the biology professor about how long it should take before his two prize bulls, which have been kept exclusively together in a holding pen, will begin producing a prize herd of cattle. The bewildered professor would probably look at him with a blank stare as he tries to explain that the two bulls will never produce any calves because they are both males and therefore cannot reproduce. It is not natural for bulls, prize specimens though they may be, to create any offspring together because their bodies are not designed to function together in that manner; it's just not normal! However, the biology professor assures the bewildered young man that this should not deter the hopeful bull breeder, as there is a way to correct the problem.

The dilemma was that this young graduate rancher had mistakenly reasoned, based on the American Psychiatric Association's 1973 reclassification of homosexuality as normal, that the same logic could be applied to animal breeding. Applying this concept—without realistically achieving the desired result—to animal breeding would require the American Biological Association to radically change historically held beliefs. To do that, they would first have to find a group of highly respected, predisposed, progressive-minded biologists in positions of authority and have them vote on the nature of cattle reproduction. The ABA could then declare that sexual encounters between bulls are perfectly normal and that such behavior should be considered acceptable. You could also vote in the same manner for cows to pair up with each other, if that is your preference. It is as simple as that! It worked in 1973 for homosexuals with the American Psychiatric Association, so it should work even better now, given how much more enlightened we are today. Who would have ever thought that a group of highly esteemed homosexual biology professors, by taking a simple vote, would be able to redefine nature? But let us not stop there and think about how we could advance all the sciences, à la the new psychological voting method, which we can now apply toward curing such fearful diseases as cancer! Or what parent with a child who has Down Syndrome, an affliction that alters a person's physical, mental, and social development, would not love to be able to make them normal by a vote, too? There is no end to what this holistic, democratic, healing approach to medicine can accomplish! It is truly a medical boon for mankind. We are now told that men can become pregnant! Could the young farmer's prize bulls be far behind?[39] However, we should be forewarned that once we begin redefining the obvious to serve an agenda, there is no limit to how far this can go. In 1991, members of the American Psychiatric Association proposed that it be improper to use heterosexual bias in language and that using heterosexual references should be avoided.

Neal Hardin, holder of a Theological Master of Arts degree, writes:

> Pronouns are small words with big implications. When signifying persons, pronouns often carry other characteristics of the people they refer to, like number and gender. And until recently, most people understood gender to be binary (male or female). But now, an ever-growing list of pronouns have become expressions of one's self-proclaimed identity, a claim that proponents insist everyone must affirm—or else.
>
> Some people have lost their jobs or been threatened with termination for refusing to use certain pronouns, which

---

[39] Jamie Eske. (Updated Aug. 10, 2026). Can men become pregnant: What to know. In *www.medicalnewstoday.com*. Transgender men and Transmasculine can whttps://www.medicalnewstoday.com/articles/can-men-become-pregnant

they believe inherently and unavoidably misrepresent a person's true nature. In other cases, people have been banned from common or public spaces—all because they believe what has been obvious to human society for thousands of years: that a man is a man and a woman is a woman. Writing for the majority, Justice Brett Kavanaugh stated that Title IX permits separate teams based on biological sex because of the "inherent physical differences between biological men and biological women."

Along this line of thought, the Supreme Court on June 20, 2026, upheld state laws that ban transgender athletes from participating in girls' and women's sports.[40]

The Title IX regulations allowed separate sports teams precisely because of the inherent physical differences between biological men and biological women," according to the majority opinion authored by Justice Brett Kavanaugh and joined by five other ideologically conservative justices.

---

[40] Lawrence Hurley, "Supreme Court Upholds Bans on Transgender Athletes in Girls' and Women's Sports," NBC News, June 30, 2026, https://www.nbcnews.com/politics/supreme-court/supreme-court-upholds-state-transgender-sports-bans-rcna261384.

> The decision partly answers questions that have sparked a number of civil rights investigations and lawsuits against states and districts, initiated both by the U.S. Department of Education and parents who say transgender student inclusion discriminates against and jeopardizes the safety of cisgender (the sex they were born with) girls.
>
> It also allows state laws separating athletics based on "biological sex" — which have proliferated in over half of the nation in recent years — to remain in place.[41]

However, as of August 12, 2026, some national professional sports still include men posing as girls. Here is an example from the National Basketball Association (WNBA):

> "Today's meeting covered a wide range of topics, including ongoing discussions on transgender athletes and the continued hate and vitriol directed at players online. We will continue to engage all league stakeholders in the coming weeks and months. We will approach these important conversations thoughtfully and in alignment with the values of our league. There are no immediate

[41] Naaz Modan, "Supreme Court Says Schools Can Separate Athletics Based on 'Biological Sex,'" K-12 Dive, June 30, 2026, https://www.k12dive.com/news/supreme-court-says-schools-can-separate-athletics-based-on-biological-sex/824083/.

eligibility matters affecting the WNBA and we strongly denounce the bad-faith efforts to use these topics to demean or marginalize others."[42]

Another unforeseen consequence of redefining an abnormality by a vote is that the same could be done to anything traditionally considered normal behavior. For example, praying to an invisible God and believing that God hears you is crazy, but believing that cryptocurrency exists in cyberspace and has value is normal—yet both require faith in the invisible! The danger of simply voting to change what is and is not normal is that some practices we consider normal today could just as easily be reclassified as abnormal tomorrow. Take, for instance, Christianity. Based on what we just discussed regarding praying to an invisible God and having faith in an invisible cryptocurrency, the supporters of homosexuality could make Christianity—or any religion for that matter—become a mental disorder and allow the person of faith to be confined indefinitely in an asylum without the benefit of a trial in a court of law. That would open a whole new area of intimidation and the silencing of Pastors, Rabbis, Christian

---

[42] Katie Barnes and Multiple Authors. "WNBA Task Force Discusses Transgender Athletes amid Furor." *ESPN*, ESPN Internet Ventures, www.espn.com/wnba/story/_/id/49594734/wnba-task-force-discusses-transgender-athletes-amid-furor. Accessed 15 Aug. 2026.

counselors, Christian psychologists, and other dissenters regarding the questioning of same-sex attractions being normal, based on their religion or any legitimate scientific observation. However, think about this in the spirit of George Orwell's book 1984,[43] and the Thinkpol also known as the Thought Police, who sought out and punished thought crimes. Does today's "hate crimes" sound familiar?

To be honest, we must conclude that both actual science and the pseudoscience of Psychology/Psychiatry are constantly in flux. While the Bible is not a science book, it does contain science and the best counsel for the study of the human soul.

We have focused on the "science of sexuality" here because it is the most controversial area of psychiatry that most people are familiar with today. Still, we acknowledge there are other subtle areas of human conflict that are equally important and trouble people's souls. Freud, an atheist,[44] coined the term psychology by combining two Greek words, *psyche,* which is the human "soul," and *ology,* which translates to mean the "study

---

[43] George Orwell, *1984* (1949; reprint, Boston: Houghton Mifflin Harcourt, 2013).

[44] Mark Edmundson, "Religion and Faith - Sigmund Freud - Atheism," *The New York Times*, September 9, 2007, https://www.nytimes.com/2007/09/09/magazine/09wwln-lede-t.html.

of," together they form a word that means "the study of the soul." Which is the better way to discern and counsel the human soul, using an atheist's contrived philosophy or the Bible? This is just another example of psychology/psychiatry's shortfall as a bona fide science; one may call it political correctness, compassion, well-meaning tolerance, or just plain ignorance—maybe—but not a science.

One could hardly be faulted for concluding that a group of people who make up only a small percentage in the single digits of the population had cleverly manipulated themselves into the perception of normality and acceptance.

In the above scenario, we have seen—regarding science and the psychology of sexuality—through an unemotional expose' of how homosexuality has become an exercise in *reductio ad absurdum.*[45]

---

[45]*Reductio ad absurdum* (Latin for "reduction to the absurd"), also known as *argumentum ad absurdum* (Latin: argument from absurdity), is a common form of argument which seeks to demonstrate that a statement is true by showing that a false, untenable, or absurd result follows from its denial, or in turn to demonstrate that a statement is false by showing that a false, untenable, or absurd result follows from its acceptance. <http://en.wikipedia.org/wiki/Reductio_ad_absurdum> accessed: 29,March 2013

CHAPTER FOUR

COULD HOMOSEXUALITY BE GENETIC?

Many scientists are searching for a genetic justification to explain homosexuality as an inherited phenomenon that cannot be reversed or criticized. Therefore, we should not be surprised to learn that some scientists are attempting to justify homosexual behavior as being normal. What we have here is basically establishing a conclusion and then looking for the evidence to prove it.

Fundamental science typically begins with the basics and follows whatever leads manifest themselves—and wherever they may take them—without being unnaturally influenced by a preconceived outcome.

In an article by Larry Thompson, Senior Director of Communications, Johnson & Johnson Office of the Chief

Medical Officer at the National Institutes of Health, Bethesda, MD, titled *More Evidence that Homosexuality is Genetic,* " *Thompson* discusses how scientists are looking for a "gay gene."[46] Thompson begins his observations in this article by addressing an experiment in which "A DNA transplant made these male fruit flies turn away from females. What does that say about the origins of homosexuality?" Of course, as provocative as this may sound—male fruit flies no longer desire to mate with female fruit flies but with other males—the male's DNA was unnaturally *manipulated* through an event (transplantation) that does not occur in nature. That is no different than a human male becoming a *eunuch* through castration.

After a detailed explanation of how the scientist manipulated the fruit flies, resulting in their unique behavior—a behavior not observed in the wild, as far as we know—Thompson concludes:

> Scientists caution against jumping to conclusions about the meaning of the NIH studies. To complicate the picture, some of the work shows that the environment, along with genetics, influences sexual behavior. In one experiment, a

---

[46]Larry Thompson. "SEARCH FOR A GAY GENE." *Time*. Time Inc., 12 June 1995. Web. 05 Aug. 2014.

small group of "straight" flies was mixed with a larger group of genetically altered "gay" flies....In fruit flies, and certainly in humans, sexual orientation is just not a simple matter. And no amount of scientific research is going to change that fact of life.[47]

If homosexuality were genetic, it would require a *mutation* in the genetic makeup. Mutations, by their very nature, are almost impossible to be passed on. To put it simply, specific molecules within the cell recognize improper coding in the DNA strand, and remove the mutant factors, then replace them with correctly coded ones. They do this by turning off specific malfunctioning genes and replacing them with the correct molecular genetic sequencing.[48]

If there is an unchecked mutated "homosexual gene" passed on in an otherwise heterosexual biological entity and it follows its predisposed primary function, which is not to reproduce itself, then that individual biological entity would die fulfilling its prime directive, which is not to procreate, thereby allowing that

---

[47] Ibid.

[48] Mary AnnClark, Jung Choi, and Matthew Douglas. 2018. "22.6 – DNA Repair." Biology 110, Pennsylvania State University. OpenStax Biology 2nd Edition. March 5, 2018. https://psu.pb.unizin.org/biol110/chapter/dna-repair/.

non-replicating gene to die with it. At best, in a higher biological organism such as a human, this type of gene could be passed on only to the second, or possibly third, generation, and only by exerting sheer willpower against its predisposed nature—a commitment not easily accomplished. In order for an actual genetic homosexual to participate in a heterosexual manifestation, it would require the homosexual to go against their genetic predisposition, presumably by being manipulated through outside pressures such as social acceptance, etc.

However, having said this, it would be almost impossible for that genetic predisposition (a predisposition containing a prime directive not to replace itself) to survive one or two generations before becoming completely extinct. For this rare condition, consisting of 1 to 2% of the population,[49] such predisposed genetic mutations would have disappeared thousands of years ago if they were genetic.

The amazing scientific fact is that the natural process of genetic development tends to be self-correcting. When new breeds are developed, they are always created in a controlled or isolated environment that we call a breeding environment. On the

---

[49] Volokh, Eugene. "What Percentage of the U.S. Population Is Gay, Lesbian or Bisexual?" *The Washington Post*, 15 July 2014.

Galápagos Islands, the unique creatures there were adaptations caused by their natural confinement on those islands.[50] Nevertheless, the various breeds produced are always within the *same* species, and *no new* genetic information is added; indeed, new species within a species are developed by the *loss* of genetic information and not by the addition of genetic information (i.e., the original canine wolf begets a Saint Bernard, and the miniature poodle alike. "Dogs and wolves living today derive from a shared ancient wolf population that lived alongside woolly mammoths."[51] If one were to collect and interbreed the various dog species, the genetic pool would be restored, resulting in a dog that resembled its original wolf-like ancestor.

In light of all that we have learned, perhaps the scientific medical community can now tackle a cure for cancer, as they did for homosexuality, by taking a vote and making cancerous cells that divide faster than their sister cells considered normal. Once this cell abnormality is voted on and passed, there should

---

[50] Jyoti Baid, "Galápagos Wildlife: A Visual Journey into Evolution's Playground," Story at Every Corner, December 25, 2022, https://storyateverycorner.com/galapagos-incredible-wildlife/.

[51] Audrey T. Lin and Logan Kistler, review of *Thousands of genomes reveal the wild wolf genes in most dogs' DNA*, Si.edu, November 24, 2025, https://www.si.edu/stories/your-dog-little-wolfy.

no longer be a need to treat cancer cells because, as we showed, they would now be deemed just as "normal" as their counterparts. Democracy in medicine is a wonderful thing.

CHAPTER FIVE

HOW DOES A HOMOSEXUAL COUPLE BEING MARRIED HARM HETEROSEXUAL MARRIAGES AND SOCIETY AT LARGE?

A survey of Marriage 101 is required to understand why civilized societies have needed an institution for heterosexual (man and woman) marriage. First, in all societies and religious systems throughout recorded history, marriage has been sanctioned for obvious reasons. When a man and a woman engage in sexual relations, it is usually just a matter of time before a woman becomes pregnant. Specific rules and restrictions had to be created to control this strong human drive. As we discussed in Chapter 2, when considering the painful birthing experience that women go through to bring a new life into this world, there had to be a drive, or stimulation, if you prefer, to deliver a very pleasurable experience in order to entice a woman to engage in sexual behavior, the aftermath of which could result in something that could become very painful. Both men and women alike, engaging in sexual behavior upon reaching a climax, experience the release of endorphins in the brain that act like the release of an incredible narcotic drug.[52] Needless to say, such an activity becomes habit-forming very quickly. There is a unique sex hormone called oxytocin, which is a powerful neuropeptide known as the "love hormone." It is a bonding hormone that allows mothers of newborn babies to see their tiny baby as beautiful, where others may not be so inclined. It is also a precursor to marriage in the sense that when people view sex in the traditional way, it also stimulates a bonding effect for a couple. This effect draws a man and a woman closer together, especially if they have never had a sexual relationship before. It really tightens marriage bonds between heterosexual couples. However, when a person begins to have multiple sex partners, the bonding effect weakens, and eventually it becomes harder for that person to form stable or long-lasting commitments without straying and having sex with partners outside their current relationship. Think about it like this: oxytocin is like duct tape. You tape the hands of two people with the tape, but after peeling it off, it

---

[52] Review of *D.O.S.E. : The brain's happy chemicals, explained.*, Khiron Clinics, January 11, 2020, https://khironclinics.com/blog/the-brains-happy-chemicals-explained/.

doesn't stick as strongly when reattached, and after peeling it off and reattaching it many times, it loses its ability to hold, just like oxytocin reacts with multiple sex partners! Of course, this does seem like oxytocin was intended to ensure marriage by what some would call a creator, but whether it, along with sex, is a plan of God or not is not the focus here, but rather the observable science and how it applies across the board of sexually active people, straight or not.

Second, casual sexual encounters without responsibility, especially for men, had to be enforced. When females past the age of puberty are allowed—through uncontrolled fornication—to produce babies continually—without the support of a family structure—it not only results in overpopulation—but also leaves a woman and her children five times more likely to live in poverty, starvation, and despair.
Humans realized long ago that when restraints are placed on sexual activity, society becomes more stable. Because the family structure is the foundational unit upon which civilized society is built, its destruction will soon lead to society's collapse.

Research has recently concluded—predictably—that men and women are different, physically, psychologically, and emotionally (notwithstanding the latest psychobabble's preposterous claim that there are over 70 sexes)[53]. Men tend to be more physical, domineering, and protective of their mate, while women tend to be more sensitive and nurturing. The bottom line of heterosexual couples serves the natural progression, which is the purpose and need for replenishing a country's population as the older generation dies. This is why countries that have allowed abortions are now facing the need to bring emigrants into their countries to bolster their infrastructure and keep their citizenry from becoming overpopulated with the elderly, a situation that can lead to a nation being overthrown by a younger, more vigorous country.

Religion, including Pagan or otherwise, has played an essential role in the development of the family. Acknowledging that the sex drive is something society must deal with, some form of regulation becomes necessary to prevent it from getting out of control; therefore, a society tries to discourage casual sexual encounters outside of a socially approved institution. Sex outside of marriage has been frowned upon by societies for millennia, yet societies also realize that people will sooner or later engage in sexual activity. Thus, both religions and

---

[53] Shaziya Allarakha, MD. "How Many Genders Are There? All 72 Genders List." *MedicineNet*, MedicineNet, 9 Feb. 2024, <www.medicinenet.com/what_are_the_72_other_genders/article.htm.>

societies developed the sanction (approval) of an institution that allows couples to engage in sex, which produces babies, but producing those babies with society's approval, as well as the approval of their religious system. That institution is known as marriage.

Because homosexuality never produces babies, such a societal sanction is not necessary. The problem with homosexual marriage is that it is a dead end and can do nothing to replace the elderly as they die. Legitimizing homosexual marriage demeans, cheapens, and negates the real purpose and reasons for heterosexual marriage, which, as we saw, is the protection of the family structure and the children it produces. One example is when marriage between a man and a woman was thought of as "Holy Matrimony"; yet today it's been reduced to "A reality show that follows singles yearning for a life-long partnership as they agree to a provocative proposal: getting legally married to a stranger the moment they first meet."[54] After the show is over and the couple finds they really don't like

---

[54] Krutika Mallikarjuna, "Married at First Sight Season 18: Meet the Couples," Netflix Tudum, May 14, 2026, https://www.netflix.com/tudum/articles/married-at-first-sight-season-18-release-date-news.

each other, they can always get a divorce. The show is so popular that as of 2026, it has had 20 seasons!

While we do not desire to be overly tedious on this subject, we must look at the unforeseen effect that homosexual marriage is having on today's society. Marriage and the family structure have traditionally been vital parts of civilization. Yet today—to the detriment of today's society—some heterosexual youth will bypass what to them has become merely a formality in the shadow of homosexual marriage, and that marriage is nothing more than the approval of couples having sex, so they choose simply to hook up or shack up without any real commitment. While revisionists and the WOKE media deny this, the U.S. Census Bureau does show that after the Supreme Court of the United States, on June 26, 2015—ignoring all precedent as well as Congress's prerogative to make laws—legalized homosexual marriage, and as a result we now see that, "For Young Adults, Cohabitation Is Up, Marriage Is Down."[55]

We have been watching this phenomenon slowly manifest itself, beginning in the 1960s. As the homosexual agenda picked up influence in the 1970s, more and more of America's

---

[55] Benjamin Gurrentz, "Living with an Unmarried Partner Now Common for Young Adults," Census.gov, November 15, 2018, https://www.census.gov/library/stories/2018/11/cohabitation-is-up-marriage-is-down-for-young-adults.html.

youth began to forgo sanctioning their relationships through marriage. To them, sex of all kinds had become more of an enjoyable pastime rather than a commitment. With the onset of 2015, on June 26, the Supreme Court, in a 5-to-4 decision, legalized marriage between a man and a man or a woman and a woman, bringing what was once considered by many to be the sacredness of marriage into an exercise in futility. Now we can even see homosexual marriages being performed at our nation's most prestigious military institutions, West Point,[56] and the United States Naval Academy, Annapolis![57] Thus, the foundation of what was once the cornerstone of America and the bedrock of all societies was no longer valued, allowing for the decline in America's once-celebrated moral fabric to begin its downward spiral.

Looking back through the prism of history on what has been the moral norm of most societies throughout the ages, and despite revisionist debunking of the words of a very celebrated man,

---

[56] Paul Singer. "West Point Chapel Hosts First Same-Sex Marriage" *USA TODAY* WEB (Dec.1, 2012) https://www.usatoday.com/story/news/nation/2012/11/30/ west-point-same-sex-marriage/1738665/

[57] "U.S. Naval Academy Hosts First Same-Sex Wedding for Maryland Couple" NBC NEWS WEB (May 10, 2014) David Bucher, a 49-year-old Academy graduate who works at the Pentagon, and partner Bruce Moats, 50, tied the knot. (May 10, 2014) https://www.nbcnews.com/news/us-news/u-s-naval-academy-hosts-first-same-sex-wedding-maryland-n102276

this passage attributed to Alexis de Tocqueville from the time of America's *Age of Revolution* (1775 to 1825), still holds true:

> Not until I went into the churches of America and heard her pulpits flame with righteousness did I understand the secret of her genius and power. America is great because she is good, and if America ever ceases to be good, she will cease to be great.

Families are made up of couples with children, but the only way homosexual couples can have children is through adoption or artificial insemination, both of which require the natural use of a woman's egg impregnated by a man's sperm. Heather may have two mommies, but she has no dad. Regardless of all the arguments to the contrary, a man can never be a mom, and a mom can never be a dad. Therefore, as we have seen, the institution of marriage was created as a societal approval of sexual activity between men and women that often creates babies. Homosexual couples do not produce babies; consequently, homosexual marriage is an oxymoron forced on this society by the nonlaw-making entity of the Supreme Court of the United States. Constitutionally, it is only the Congress of the United States that is permitted to create laws.

Nevertheless, as we have stated, by normalizing Homosexual marriage—marriage as an institution—becomes meaningless with the predictable results of heterosexual couples simply living together—a phenomenon that has become the norm in our society and is portrayed that way in many television and motion picture shows both here and abroad.

No Longer Is the Issue Just Homosexuals, But Transgenders as Well

A new phenomenon, which we touched on earlier, is the rapid increase in schoolchildren from kindergarten upward who think of themselves as the opposite sex from the one they were born with. That is called transgender or transitioning away from what you physically are toward the sex you are not. At the end of our final Chapter 6, we learn that the Daughters of the American Revolution (DAR) now allow men, pretending to also be daughters, to join that once-prestigious organization. Most people are aware that if they really desire to change their sexual appearance, they can take advantage of hormone shots and have cosmetic sex-change surgery. While this might accomplish the desired outward physical effect of a woman looking like a man or a man looking like a woman, they still have the XX female or XY male chromosomes that determine their true sex, which cannot be changed. Therefore, what they were at conception is unchangeable except for outward appearances. Sadly, these people are only deluding themselves into believing they are someone they are not. One argument is that they were born that way; therefore, they are really a man or woman trapped in a woman's or man's body. This strawman argument is easy to set up (a strawman argument is like a scarecrow made out of straw, which is easy to prop up and easy to knock down). It is a way of attacking an opponent's position by twisting the facts and making it easier to discredit); however, in light of the existence of male and female chromosomes, as we have just shown, this strawman argument can just as easily be knocked down too. Therefore, like it or not, this now becomes a religious argument because if one were to say, "I'm a woman, trapped in a man's body," what is the female entity that you believe you are, that is trapped in a man's body, supposed to be? By that very line of reasoning, it would have to be the spirit of a woman trapped in a man's body. As for us (you and I), we cannot force our religious beliefs on anyone, much less the public school system; but the school system itself is forcing the religion of transgenderism on heterosexual schoolchildren. This thinking has now allowed a male student who claims he is a girl to shower with the girls, use the girls' locker room, and even use their school restrooms and attempt to compete in girls' sports.

Another unforeseen consequence of the unscientific APA's official Diagnostic and Statistical Manual of Psychiatric Disorders vote normalizing homosexuality is that now homosexuals who want to be a woman so they can enjoy sex with men (transgenderism) has also spilled over into our classrooms, public restrooms, and business establishments. Another outgrowth is the mainstreaming of the homosexual agenda in entertainment, commercials, and children's comic books. Marvel Comics now features seven superheroes who are transgender and a new Captain America who is a homosexual! Not to be outdone, DC Comics made Superman become homosexual as well. "The Obama-Biden Administration had appointed 250 homosexuals, more than all known LGBTQ appointments of other presidential administrations combined." Not to be outdone, when Joe Biden became president, he created even more in his administration![58]

---

[58] "LGBTQ Appointments in the Biden-Harris Administration." *LGBTQ+ Victory Institute*, 27 Feb. 2024, victoryinstitute.org/programs/political-appointments-program/lgbtq-appointments-in-the-biden-harris-administration/.

A PROPHETIC WORD FROM THE PROGRESSIVE LEFT:

The late Progressive prophet, Daniel Patrick Moynihan (March 16, 1927-March 26, 2003), a Diplomat, scientist, and Democrat Senator from New York, argued that when a country can no longer deal with a certain level of deviant (abnormal, aberrant, different) behavior, it might decide to lower the standards. Quoting Kai T. Erikson,[59] Sen. Moynihan stated:

> ...the amount of deviant behavior in American society has increased beyond the levels the community can "afford to recognize" and that, accordingly, we have been redefining deviancy so as to exempt much conduct previously stigmatized, and also quietly raising the "normal" level in categories where behavior is now abnormal by any earlier standard.

Yet in 1973, despite arguing the fact that there was no scientific evidence supporting the claim by the homosexual lobby that homosexuality was normal, the American Psychological Association was coerced to vote quickly to delete

---

[59] Penelope Laurans, review of *Kai T. Erikson, eminent sociologist and historian of disaster*, Yale News, November 11, 2025, https://news.yale.edu/2025/11/11/kai-t-erikson-eminent-sociologist-and-historian-disaster.

homosexuality from the *Diagnostic and Statistical Manual of Psychiatric Disorders*. Thus—by a single vote—homosexuality became medically approved as normal behavior.

CHAPTER SIX

WHERE WE ARE NOW

As we suggested earlier, when a previously established standard is altered to accommodate normalization of its counterpart, there can be unforeseen consequences. Earlier, we showed how, with a simple vote, homosexuality became normal. Could it also be true that by a vote, people of faith could become marginalized and reclassified as abnormal[60] and subjected to confinement in an asylum against their will?

One of the unforeseen consequences of redefining homosexuality resulted in homosexual marriages and adoptions being allowed for homosexual couples, which caused the Catholic Church's Adoption Agency in America to close down. In 2009, in England, we saw the same moral conflict with

[60] Review of *Defining Abnormality: The Four D's and Cultural Context • Psychology Town*, Psychology Town, July 29, 2024, https://psychology.town/fundamentals-of-mental-health/defining-abnormality-four-ds-cultural-context/.

the Catholic Church's Adoption Agencies. However, in the United Kingdom, after a period of time, some Catholic Adoption Agencies recanted, and about half decided to comply with man's law rather than God's Law.[61]

The next step in this progression of traditional moral decay led to a redefinition of what constitutes a typical family and a normal marriage. After spending a few hours on social media since the Supreme Court's ruling on same-sex marriage (ignoring historical judicial precedent), the most often asked rhetorical question from the Left has been, "How does a gay couple's marriage hurt your heterosexual marriage, and how does it harm society?" That's another straw man argument . To begin with, all weddings should be a gay event in the traditional sense. Our wedding was a gay (lighthearted, happy) event. Thankfully, I have never been to a wedding that was a sad event.

---

[61]Charman, Rachel. "Catholic Agencies Turn on Gay Adoption Rights as Exemption Period Runs out." *PinkNews*. N.p., 2 Jan. 2009. Web. 02 Aug. 2015. Catholic agencies turn on gay adoption rights as exemption period runs out 50% of the Catholic adoption agencies that threatened to close if forced to work with gay couples have adopted the new equality law. 11 agencies were given a 21 month exemption period from the Equality Act in April 2007, which forbade discrimination in the provision of good and services on the grounds of sexuality. The exemption period ran out at the start of the new year. Of those 11 agencies, five have changed their position and will now comply with the laws, whilst one is to close, and two are still seeking exemption, BBC News reports.

Progressives love to redefine terms, and if we, those who are traditionalists or conservative, disagree, they are labeled using race, sex, and/or religion with words like "bigot" or "phobic" (a phobia is an *unnatural* fear of something) tacked on the end for the sake of intimidation.

Presumably, when one asks a rhetorical question, it is usually framed as a question that demands a negative response, not as a statement that could be answered in the affirmative. An example of this type of answer to a rhetorical question could be, "I don't know" or "Who can say?"

How do we respond? The Left is convinced most Conservatives are discriminating against homosexuals, but they are actually reacting to something that will have more significant implications than initially conceived of, and some negative consequences we won't know for a very long time. Consider some immediate implications of the ruling allowing homosexual marriages. Two things may appear: many churches and religious groups will provide the most significant pushback by fighting for their constitutional rights (as the Bible condemns the practice of homosexuality), and some already have caved and accommodated gay marriages.[62]

Previously, the law did not allow homosexuality to be tolerated. Now the law has made it so it must be elevated and considered equally acceptable as normal—again,[63] all by a vote from unelected individuals. While not a complete list, what follows are more unforeseen consequences of redefining what is normal and what is not using bullet points:

- In many public schools, they have allowed boys to use the girls' bathrooms if a boy claims he is a girl "trapped" in a boy's body. Add this to girls playing sports that only boys used to play, so they share locker rooms and showers. The blurring of the sex lines has now become a national issue.[64]
- In our nation's public schools, teachers are told to begin grooming children from pre-school age upward, instructing the children about transgenderism and that a boy may not

---

[62] HRS Staff, review of *Reformation Day: Protestant Christians Embrace LGBTQ Diversity*, HRC, October 31, 2017.

[63] Justia, "Bowers v. Hardwick, 478 U.S. 186 (1986)," Justia Law, 2019, https://supreme.justia.com/cases/federal/us/478/186/.

[64] *U.S. Department of Education Opens Three New Investigations into Michigan School Districts for Alleged Title IX Violations*, U.S. Department of Education, June 18, 2026, https://www.ed.gov/about/news/press-release/us-department-of-education-opens-three-new-investigations-michigan-school-districts-alleged-title-ix-violations.

really be a boy and a girl may not really be a girl. Many schools have even shown these impressionable little children pornographic material/books designed for small children to be indoctrinated with as well as exposing them to lewd acts of actual scantily clad transgender men dressed as women performing in front of the children.[65]

- Free speech is already beginning to be marginalized.[66]
- Traditional moralists will be branded as bigoted, homophobic, and anti-social like the Utah National Guardsman who was reprimanded for saying same sex marriage is a "mockery of God." He appealed, but a U.S. District Judge dismissed the charge made by a "Mormon who in 2012 used his military email account to object to an official at West Point about a same-sex wedding taking place at the academy's chapel."[67]

---

[65] *Sarah Parshall Perry, "Parents Are Fed Up With Public Schools Secretly Transitioning Children," The Heritage Foundation, March 28, 2023, https://www.heritage.org/gender/commentary/parents-are-fed-public-schools-secretly-transitioning-children.*

[66] Aniceto Masferrer, review of *The Decline of Freedom of Expression and Social Vulnerability in Western democracy, International Journal for the Semiotics of Law - Revue Internationale de Sémiotique Juridique* 36 (March 12, 2023), https://doi.org/10.1007/s11196-023-09990-1.

[67] Chris Johnson, "Court Upholds Reprimand for Airman Who Opposed Gay Wedding," Washington Blade: LGBTQ News, Politics, LGBTQ Rights, Gay News, October 16, 2015, https://www.washingtonblade.com/2015/10/16/court-upholds-reprimand-for-airman-who-opposed-gay-wedding/.

- While the State does not mandate churches' beliefs, pastors could still be censored for teaching so-called "hate speech" in their sermons when they talk about the Bible and homosexuality; however, with this ruling, they could also lose their tax-exempt status.[68]
- Military chaplains: Because marrying homosexuals is now the Law of the Land chaplains could be disciplined or even lose their commission and all military benefits if they refuse to marry homosexual couples.[69] We have seen such marriages at West Point and Annapolis[70].
- Churches meeting in public schools cannot teach that homosexuality is unnatural for fear of being denied the school as their meeting place.
- Parents' religious beliefs will become marginalized through the public educational system, and children will be turned against their parents and their religion.

---

[68] Josh Sanburn, review of *Houston Pastors Find Themselves in City's Crosshairs*, TIME, October 17, 2014, https://time.com/3514166/houston-pastors-sermons-subpoenaed/.

[69] "Military Chaplains Raise Gay Marriage Concerns," Prairie Public (Prairie Public NewsRoom, May 13, 2012), https://news.prairiepublic.org/2012-05-13/military-chaplains-raise-gay-marriage-concerns.

[70] NBC News, "U.S. Naval Academy Hosts First Same-Sex Wedding for Maryland Couple," NBC News, May 10, 2014, https://www.nbcnews.com/news/us-news/u-s-naval-academy-hosts-first-same-sex-wedding-maryland-n102276.

- Christian psychologists/psychiatrists, biblical counselors, doctors, and nurses could be fined or jailed if they try to help homosexuals leave that lifestyle.
- Private schools could lose government funding and accreditation if they go against the law; consequently, they will be accused of encouraging bigoted attitudes against a legal activity.
- School teachers could be forced to not only endorse and teach homosexuality against their religious beliefs but could be socially marginalized or financially penalized and lose their government (public school) jobs.
- With the legalization of homosexual marriage, children will realize that if a man and a man—or a woman and a woman—or a man and a woman can be married, there is nothing special about marriage. Marriage causes problems when you want to break up. After all, it is now only a formality and has nothing to do with making babies—so just live together and avoid all the problems of divorce.
- In 2014 California replaced the supposed outdated and biased words in the Family Code from "husband" and "wife"

to the gender-neutral word, "spouse," to accommodate same-sex marriage.[71] Expect that to happen in more states.

- Nude parades and simulated sex acts conducted in public with men, women and children watching.[72]
- We are seeing more medical transmissions for sex changes regarding children.[73] Recently on Newsmax, a speaker observed that if I were a doctor and a child asked me to cut off his arms and I did, I would be jailed. But if a child asked me to change his sex and I cut off his penis, that would be alright!
- As a newly court-sanctioned minority group, any discrimination against homosexuals becomes an issue for employers, religious organizations, housing, or public accommodation issues.

A noted Civil Rights Attorney—Richard McLellan—from Michigan, made this observation:

---

[71] "California Senate Bill 1306," LEGISCAN, accessed July 8, 2026, https://legiscan.com/CA/text/SB1306/id/966850.

[72] Todd Starnes. "July. 'a Giant Public Orgy.' Reporters Sickened by Gay Sex Acts during Pride Parade." *Todd Starnes*, 1 July 2024,< www.toddstarnes.com/crime/a-giant-public-orgy-reporters-sickened-by-gay-sex-acts-during-pride-parade/>
Todd Starnes is an award-winning journalist, best-selling author, and radio host also appearing on various news programs including Hannity.

[73] Michael Katz, "Gender Dysphoria, Use of Puberty Blockers, Surgeries Rise in US." *Newsmax*, Newsmax Media, Inc., 20 Dec. 2022, www.newsmax.com/newsfront/gender-dysphoria-minors/2022/12/19/id/1101160/.

However, if the firing, denial of housing or refusal of public accommodations was based only on the person being gay or lesbian, that would remain legal.

If you have a wedding chapel that you hold out to the public to rent for weddings, can you deny a gay couple that wants to get married there?" he asked. "I would say no you cannot."

- More far-reaching results on the normalization of homosexuality can be found in the Boy Scouts of America (BSA). This organization was forced to rename itself *Scouting America* on February 8, 2025, after suffering a great backlash and financial losses due to its caving to the accommodation of homosexual Scout Masters in its ranks. To reinvent itself, it now claims it is more reflective of a modern, inclusive approach to youth programs and, for that reason, has dropped the name "Boy Scouts of America" from its profile. More likely, the truth is that, because of declining numbers, BSA sought to rebuild its ranks by allowing girls to fill the empty spots left by Boy Scout dropouts.

The trouble began when it was pressured to start allowing gay youth to join on January 1, 2014. Shortly after, the organization lifted its ban on openly gay adult leaders and volunteers, which officially went into effect on July 27, 2015[74]

Of course, today the revamped organization has no resemblance to the one founded in 1910 by W. D. Boyce, which had involved over 130 million Americans in its programs over the past century. Yet despite the lawsuits and being forced into bankruptcy, the new pro-homosexual organization is mounting a positive campaign and spin to cover its problems. According to the Liberal Public Broadcasting website:

> When it sought bankruptcy protection in 2020, the Boy Scouts of America had been named in about 275 lawsuits, and told insurers it was aware of another 1,400 claims.
>
> Last year [2023] a federal judge upheld the $2.4 billion bankruptcy plan allowing the organization to keep operating while compensating more than 80,000 men who filed claims saying they were sexually abused as children and teen scouts.[75]

- In concluding our bullet observations, we will reveal an unforeseen consequence caused by the vote on normalizing

[74]Justin Sullivan. (2015, July 28). *Boy scouts of America lifts decades-old ban on gay troop leaders*. ABCnews. https://www.abc.net.au/news/2015-07-28/boy-scouts-lift-ban-on-gay-scoutmasters/6653268

[75] Here's why the Boy Scouts of America are rebranding. (2024). In *PBS NewsHour*. https://www.pbs.org/newshour/nation/heres-why-the-boy-scouts-of-america-are-rebranding

homosexuality, which opened the door for men pretending to be daughters to infiltrate the children of our Founding Fathers. Those children are the Daughters of the American Revolution (DAR), which was founded in 1890 by godly women whose biblical motto is "God, Home and Country' believing, among other things, that marriage is to be between a man and a woman (Genesis 2:24, Matthew 19:6; Mark 10:9)!" Consider when The Daughters of the American Revolution, 11 years to the day—after SCOTUS legalized HOMOSEXUAL MARRIAGE—held a controversial vote to allow those men pretending to be daughters into the DAR on June 26, 2026.[76] Several eyewitnesses said that on Friday, June 26th, at the DAR's 135th Continental Congress in Continental Hall, Washington, D.C., they observed irregularities during the vote on whether to admit transgender individuals to the DAR. Some of those irregularities included blocking members who opposed allowing men posing as women to speak or present their concerns.

The New York Post reported:

> For a century-plus, the DAR's very name has described both who its members are and why they belong.

[76] Valerie Richardson, "Daughters of American Revolution Assembly Defeats Proposal to Block Transgender Members," The Washington Times, June 27, 2026,<,https://www.washingtontimes.com/news/2026/jun/27/daughters-american-revolution-defeats-proposal-block-transgender/>.

It's difficult to imagine a more straightforward membership standard than one rooted in genealogy and biological reality. Yet all that has now been thrown into question over what members estimate is a grand total of between *two and five transgender* members — out of 190,000 — who call themselves "Transdaughters."

The voting process itself only deepened the divide. The congress' initial vote was scotched [scrapped] before it was counted, when opponents of the measure claimed to have seen evidence of cheating....Again and again, American institutions have discovered that appeasing ideological activists while ignoring the wishes of their core constituency is a losing strategy.

The customers leave, donors disappear, volunteers stop volunteering.

The institution slowly hollows itself out from within. Yet again and again, left-leaning leaders fall for the same trap.

There's a bitter irony in how an organization created to honor the sacrifices of America's founders chose, on the eve of the nation's 250th birthday, to jeopardize its own future over the wish to accommodate at most five people.[77]

[77] Bethany Mandel. 2026. "The Daughters of the American Revolution Are in Revolt — Because Trans Zealots Can't Leave ANYTHING Alone." The New York Post. June 30, 2026.

Note the bizarre coincidences regarding the date *June* 26 and the chain of events on that date. It was on *June 26*, 1891, that the Daughters of the American Revolution was formed. It was on *June 26*, 2015, that SCOTUS, by a vote, allowed for homosexual marriage; and it was on June 26, 2026, by a vote, that the DAR, through alleged threats and intimidation, condescended—like the members of the American Psychiatric Association—to allow transgender individuals access!

But that's not the end of it; in the face of overwhelming protest against allowing men pretending to be daughters into the DAR, and local chapters demanding a revote, the National Headquarters of the DAR responded by sending down a guideline on how a revote may be accomplished. It required providing an outlandish number of members for a revote to be considered. Not only did the local chapters meet that guideline but surpassed it only to be told it was not good enough. Talk about moving the field goal in mid-game!

Another slap in the face to the rank-and-file members of the Daughters of the American Revolution came on October 17, 2026, when DAR's Memorial Continental Hall, recognized as one of Washington, D.C.'s most elegant buildings, allowed a popular,

---

https://nypost.com/2026/06/29/opinion/daughters-of-the-american-revolution-revolt-because-trans-zealots-cant-leave-anything-alone/.

sexually overt transgender group to perform. This controversial group, known as "Trixie and Katya, a pair of grizzled gay ghouls exploring the cultural boundaries of modern beauty," was allowed to perform their drag queen show at DAR's beautiful and prestigious Constitution Hall, located in that building.

> The show brings their signature blend of camp humor, candid conversation, and unfiltered banter to life on stage. Expect outrageous comedy, pop culture commentary, and personal anecdotes, all delivered with their trademark chemistry [78]

Tickets for this sexually provocative performance start at $120.00 and go up to $1,351.00.[79] Trixie and Katya have partnered with PLUS1 so that $1 per ticket goes to support The Trevor Project, which provides crisis intervention and suicide prevention services for LGBTQ+ youth.[80]

We now come to the end of our bullet observations with this thought. It's a sad day indeed when a performance of this nature, which is completely opposite of the DAR's traditional values of

---

[78] "Trixie and Katya Playing at Dar Washington Dc - Bing." 2026 https://www.bing.com/search?q=trixie%20and%20katya%20playing%20at%20dar%20washington%20dc&qs=n&form=QBRE&sp=-ghc=1&lq=0&pq=trixie%20and%20katya%20playing%20at%20dar%20washington%20dc&sc=12-45&sk=&cvid=C132DD424AB44F5E93479CDE947C40AF.

[79] The Bald and The Beautiful at DAR Constitution Hall (10/17/2026) Tickets

[80] "Trixie and Katya Playing at DAR Washington DC - Bing." 2026.

"God, Home and Country," is allowed to be featured not only in our nation's capital but, arguably up until now, at the once respectable Daughters of the American Revolution venue. A venue that is inside of the DAR's block-long building, which is located only two blocks from the White House, and ranks as one of the largest buildings of its kind owned and maintained exclusively by women.[81] However, if they continue to allow men pretending to be daughters into the DAR, their claim of female ownership can no longer honestly be claimed.

As we have seen, ignoring science and relying on a consensus vote can have many consequences, in this case—without scientific documentation—normalizing homosexuality.

We should point out here that science deals in facts and not consensus. In an article for the *Harvard Journal of Law and Public Policy*, Chloe Jones, states:

Long before *Skrmetti*,[82] activists understood that to win

---

[81] "National Society Daughters of the American Revolution." 2024. Daughters of the American Revolution. October 24, 2024. https://www.dar.org/national-society/visitor-information.

[82] United States v. Skrmetti, 605 U.S. 495 (2025), is a Supreme Court case holding that a Tennessee state law banning the use of puberty blockers and hormone therapy for treating minors' gender dysphoria did not violate the Equal Protection Clause of the U.S. Constitution's Fourteenth Amendment.

the controversial legal "battle" on gender-transition treatments for minors, the medical field needed to present "a united front." Through coordinated efforts, these authoritative groups framed procedures like puberty blockers, cross-sex hormones, and surgeries such as double mastectomies as "standard medical care, supported by major medical organizations in the United States." This perceived consensus became a powerful tool in litigation, often used to argue that state-level restrictions were medically unfounded and constitutionally suspect. If states enacted laws restricting these procedures for minors, attorneys could seek injunctions, citing a "medical consensus [that] is grounded in a wealth of studies" that undermined the states' safety concerns. Indeed, after states began enacting such restrictions, opponents described the laws as extreme departures from scientific norms and even alleged that they "make it a crime for doctors to act ethically" and increase the likelihood that "some [transgender-identifying children] will die."[83] (Bracketed clarification hers.)

---

[83] "The Facade of Medical Consensus – Chloe Jones." *Harvard Journal of Law & Public Policy*, 3 June 2025, https://journals.law.harvard.edu/jlpp/the-facade-of-medical-consensus-chloe-jones/. Accessed 18 Aug. 2026.

Regardless of your position, we must insist that any organization claiming to be part of the medical community must, for the sake of the patient, always rely on science rather than politics or emotions. This is the reason that many people have accused both psychiatry and psychology of being pseudo (false) science. Rather than relying on empirical science, and by a vote declaring a sickness not to be a sickness and redefining that illness as an acceptable normal part of human reality, harms both the homosexual and the heterosexual person as well. Relying on a vote and not science may also erode the doctor-patient relationship, which is not good.

We will now close with the words of the distinguished late New York Democrat Senator, Daniel Moynihan,[84] and his famous observation, "Defining Deviancy Down."

> We deal with the epidemic by simply defining away most of the disease. We lower the threshold for what we are prepared to call normal in order to keep the volume of deviancy—[i.e.] redefined deviancy—within manageable

---

[84] Review of *Daniel Patrick Moynihan | United States senator and sociologist | Britannica*, www.britannica.com, June 26, 2026, https://www.britannica.com/biography/Daniel-Patrick-Moynihan.

> proportions....We are getting used to a lot of behavior that is not good for us.[85]

In conclusion, as we have seen—by a simple vote—the *Diagnostic and Statistical Manual of Mental Disorders* eliminated homosexuality as an abnormal malady. Therefore, if voting to normalize homosexuality is valid, we must ask the provocative question, "... wouldn't a parent with a child who has Down Syndrome, an affliction that alters a person's physical, mental, and social development, love to be able to make them normal by a vote as well? "

Perhaps Senator Moynihan exposed the motivation behind the driving force that makes something obviously unnatural seem natural. Could the LGBTQ community be pursuing an agenda? We will leave that for you to decide.

---

[85] Raspberry, William. "Defining Deviancy Down." *The Washington Post*, 28 Dec. 1992.

APPENDIX

Throughout this book, we have ended our chapters with the Psychologist logo, which incorporates the Greek trident letter "PSI," Ψ which signifies the psyche or soul, and entwined snakes on a rod, which signify healing and is also used separately for the medical profession. To explain why this emblem was created, we need to show the biblical purpose behind their logo. At the outset of this book, we informed the reader that for thousands of years, religion played a major part in sexual relationships but that while we must necessarily include religion in our research on the subject of homosexuality, we would nonetheless try to avoid being preachy in dealing with the subject of how homosexuality went from being considered a deviant and sinful behavior to becoming normalized. We explained that, for millennia, various religions, both pagan and monotheistic (belief in one God), had to deal with homosexuality, and that there was no way—to be forthright and honest—that we could avoid it. Nevertheless, while maintaining this profession as secular, both psychologists and psychiatrists find they must address religion, although in a limited manner, when dealing with this controversial subject. Therefore, to find the source of this snake-infested logo, we must revisit the Bible for an explanation of why they have serpents in their logo.

We find in Scripture that during the desert wandering of the children of Israel, many of them were being bitten by venomous snakes. So, God had Moses create brass serpents that, when looked upon, would heal the bitten Hebrews. The story goes like this:

> They (the Hebrews) traveled from Mount Hor along the route to the Red Sea, to go around Edom. But the people grew impatient on the way; they spoke against God and against Moses, and said, "Why have you brought us up out

of Egypt to die in the wilderness? There is no bread! There is no water! And we detest this miserable food!"
Then the Lord sent venomous snakes among them; they bit the people and many Israelites died. The people came to Moses and said, "We sinned when we spoke against the Lord and against you. Pray that the Lord will take the snakes away from us." So Moses prayed for the people.
The Lord said to Moses, "Make a snake and put it up on a pole; anyone who is bitten can look at it and live." So Moses made a bronze snake and put it up on a pole. Then when anyone was bitten by a snake and looked at the bronze snake, they lived. (Numbers 21:4-9, NIV)

Despite secular Psychologists and Psychiatrists[86] not being in the clergy, we like the fact that they still acknowledge the soul (which can also mean spirit[87]) in the name of their profession.

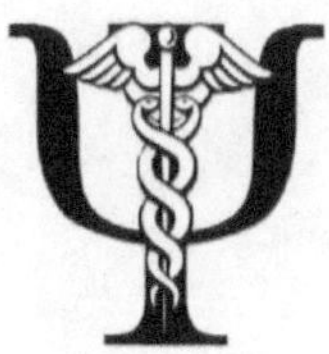

[86] Oxford Languages mid-19th century: Psychiatrists from Greek psukhē 'soul, mind' + iatreia 'healing' (from iatros 'healer')

[87] "And it came to pass, as her soul was in departing, (for she died) that she called his name Benoni: but his father called him Benjamin."(Genesis 35:18, KJV)

SOURCES CITED

Allarakha, MD, Shaziya. "How Many Genders Are There? All 72 Genders List." *MedicineNet*, MedicineNet, WEB.. 9 Feb. 2024,

American Psychiatric Association, *Diagnostic and Statistical Manual of Mental Disorders*, Text Revision Dsm-5-tr, (Washington D.C., Amer Psychiatric Pub Inc, 16 March 2022).

"Avoiding heterosexual bias in language." *American Psychologist*, vol. 46, no. 9, 1991, pp. 973–974, https://doi.org/10.1037/0003-066x.46.9.973.

Barnes, Katie, and Multiple Authors. "WNBA Task Force Discusses Transgender Athletes amid Furor." *ESPN*, ESPN Internet Ventures, www.espn.com/wnba/story/_/id/49594734/wnba-task-force-discusses-transgender-athletes-amid-furor. Accessed 15 Aug. 2026.

Beatty, R.A., *Parthenogenesis and Polyploidy in Mammalian Development (Cambridge Monographs in Experimental Biology),* First edition, (Cambridge: Cambridge University Press, 1957).

Bayer Ph.D., Ronald, *BIOETHICS Ronald Bayer, Ph.D. Bio Sketch* <https://www.publichealth.columbia.edu/profile/ronald-bayer-phd> Accessed 1 April, 2013.

_______ *Homosexuality and American Psychiatry: The Politics of Diagnosis* (Princeton: Princeton University Press, 1987).

BEHE, Michael J. *DARWIN'S BLACK BOX: THE BIOCHEMICAL CHALLENGE TO* EVOLUTION (New York, A TOUCHSTONE BOOK PUBLISHED BY SIMON & SCHUSTER, 6th Edition, 2003).

Baid, Jyoti. "Galápagos Wildlife: A Visual Journey into Evolution's Playground." Story at Every Corner, December 25, 2022. https://storyateverycorner.com/galapagos-incredible-wildlife/.

Braslow, Joel T., and Luke Messac. "Medicalization and Demedicalization — A Gravely Disabled Homeless Man with Psychiatric Illness." Edited by Scott D. Stonington, Seth M. Holmes, Helena Hansen, Jeremy A. Greene, Keith A. Wailoo, Debra Malina, Stephen Morrissey, Paul E. Farmer, and Michael G. Marmot. *New England Journal of Medicine* 379, no. 20 (November 15, 2018): 1885–88. https://doi.org/10.1056/nejmp1811623.

Bray, Chris. "Suddenly The Radical Pro-Trans Medical Organization WPATH Tells A Court That It's Just Guessing." *The Federalist*, A DIVISON OF FDRLST MEDIA, 12 Aug. 2026, thefederalist.com/2026/08/12/suddenly-the-radical-pro-trans-medical-organization-wpath-tells-a-court-that-its-just-guessing/.

Britannica Editors. “Hermaphroditism | Definition, Types, & Effects.” Encyclopædia Britannica, July 20, 1998. https://www.britannica.com/science/hermaphroditism.

Charman, Rachel. "Catholic Agencies Turn on Gay Adoption Rights as Exemption Period Runs Out." *PinkNews*. N.p., 2 Jan. 2009. Web. 02 Aug. 2015

Clark, Mary Ann , Jung Choi, and Matthew Douglas. 2018. “22.6 – DNA Repair.” Biology 110, Pennsylvania State University. OpenStax Biology 2nd Edition. March 5, 2018. https://psu.pb.unizin.org/biol110/chapter/dna-repair/.

Darwin, Charles . *On THE ORIGIN OF SPECIES or PREVISION OF FAVORED RACES IN THE STRUGGLE FOR LIFE* . (London, John Murray Publisher, 1859)

Editors of ScienceNewsToday. (2025). New Study Reveals Life on Earth May Be Far More Unlikely Than We Ever Imagined. In *Science News Today*. https://www.sciencenewstoday.org/new-study-reveals-life-on-earth-may-be-far-more-unlikely-than-we-ever-imagined

Edmundson, Mark. “Relgion and Faith - Sigmund Freud - Atheism.” *The New York Times*, September 9, 2007. https://www.nytimes.com/2007/09/09/magazine/09wwln-lede-t.html.

Ellis, Sarah Kate AKA Sarahkateellis. “Instagram.” Instagram.com, 2026.
https://www.instagram.com/p/duwfm0gdmor/.

Endsjø, Dag Ølstein. *Sex and Religion: Teachings and Taboos in the History of World Faiths* (London, UK, Reaktion Books, 15 October 2011)

Eske, Jamie. (Updated Aug. 10, 2026). Can men become pregnant: What to know. In *www.medicalnewstoday.com*. Transgender men and Transmasculine can whttps://www.medicalnewstoday.com/articles/can-men-become-pregnant

Fryer, John Ercel. "Preserving American Freedom." *Robert Palmer Knight | Exhibits.hsp.org,*

Gurrentz, Benjamin . "Living with an Unmarried Partner Now Common for Young Adults." Census.gov, November 15, 2018. https://www.census.gov/library/stories/2018/11/cohabitation-is-up-marriage-is-down-for-young-adults.html.

Laurans, Penelope. Review of *Kai T. Erikson, eminent sociologist and historian of disaster*. Yale News, November 11, 2025. https://news.yale.edu/2025/11/11/kai-t-erikson-eminent-sociologist-and-historian-disaster.

Hardin, Neil, MA, "Neal Hardin," Alliance Defending Freedom, October 28, 2025, https://adflegal.org/profile/neal-hardin/.

Here's why the Boy Scouts of America are rebranding. (2024). In *PBS NewsHour*. https://www.pbs.org/newshour/nation/heres-why-the-boy-scouts-of-america-are-rebranding

"Homosexuality and Psychology." Edited by Talk, *Wikipedia*, Wikimedia Foundation, 4 July 2024, en.wikipedia.org/wiki/Homosexuality_and_psychology.

HRS Staff. Review of *Reformation Day: Protestant Christians Embrace LGBTQ Diversity*. HRC, October 31, 2017. https://www.hrc.org/news/reformation-day-protestant-christians-embrace-lgbtq-diversity-500-years-aft.

Hurley, Lawrence. "Supreme Court Upholds Bans on Transgender Athletes in Girls' and Women's Sports," NBC News, June 30, 2026,

Institute of Medicine (US) Committee on Understanding the Biology of Sex and Gender Differences, Theresa M Wizemann, and Mary-Lou Pardue. "Every Cell Has a Sex." Nih.gov. National Academies Press (US), 2013. https://www.ncbi.nlm.nih.gov/books/NBK222291/.

Isabela Salas-Betsch, "The Economic Status of Single Mothers," Center for American Progress, August 7, 2024, https://www.americanprogress.org/article/the-economic-status-of-single-mothers/.

Jay, Karla and Allen Young (eds.). *Out of the Closets: Voices of Gay Liberation* (New York: Jove Books, 1972), 147. Under the heading *Surviving Psychotherapy,* Citing Christopher Z. Hobson.

Johnson, Chris. "Court Upholds Reprimand for Airman Who Opposed Gay Wedding." Washington Blade: LGBTQ

News, Politics, LGBTQ Rights, Gay News, October 16, 2015. https://www.washingtonblade.com/2015/1016/court-upholds-reprimand-for-airman-who-opposed-gay-wedding/.

Justia. "Bowers v. Hardwick, 478 U.S. 186 (1986)." Justia Law, 2019. https://supreme.justia.com/cases/federal/us/478/186/.

Kamman, Samantha. "Netflix's Promotion of LGBT Themes, Sexual Preferences in Kids' Shows 'Pervasive': Report." Christianpost.com. The Christian Post, December 11, 2025.

Kaspersky. "What Is Cryptocurrency and How Does It Work?" Kaspersky, 2022. https://www.kaspersky.com/resource-center/definitions/what-is-cryptocurrency.

Katz, Michael. "Gender Dysphoria, Use of Puberty Blockers, Surgeries Rise in US." *Newsmax*, Newsmax Media, Inc. Newsmax Media, Inc., 20 Dec. 2022,

Krutika Mallikarjuna. "Married at First Sight Season 18: Meet the Couples." Netflix Tudum, May 14, 2026. https://www.netflix.com/tudum/articles/married-at-first-sight-season-18-release-date-news.

Leary, Timothy Francis, (October 22, 1920--May 31, 1996) was an American psychologist and writer, known for his advocacy of psychedelic drugs

Lega, Federico. *Elgar Encyclopedia of Healthcare Management*. Cheltenham, UK: Edward Elgar Publishing, 2023.

Legacy. "John McDevitt Obituary (2007) - New York, NY - New York Times." Legacy.com. Legacy, November 22, 2007. https://www.legacy.com/us/obituaries/nytimes/name/john-mcdevitt-obituary?id=33083155.

LEGISCAN. "California Senate Bill 1306." Accessed July 8, 2026. https://legiscan.com/CA/text/SB1306/id/966850.
Bill Title: Marriage.sponsorship: Partisan Bill (Democrat 1)
Status: (Passed) 2014-07-07 - Chaptered by Secretary of State. Chapter 82, Statutes of 2014. [SB1306 Detail]

Lin, Audrey T., and Logan Kistler. Review of *Thousands of genomes reveal the wild wolf genes in most dogs' DNA*. Si.edu, November 24, 2025. https://www.si.edu/stories/your-dog-little-wolfy.

"LGBTQ Appointments in the Obama-Biden Administration." *LGBTQ+ Victory Institute*, 9 Feb. 2023

Mandel, Bethany. 2026. "The Daughters of the American Revolution Are in Revolt — Because Trans Zealots Can't Leave ANYTHING Alone." The New York Post. June 30, 2026.
https://nypost.com/2026/06/29/opinion/daughters-of-the-american-revolution-revolt-because-trans-zealots-cant-leave-anything-alone/.

Masferrer, Aniceto. Review of *The Decline of Freedom of Expression and Social Vulnerability in Western democracy. International Journal for the Semiotics of Law - Revue Internationale de Sémiotique Juridique* 36 (March 12, 2023). https://doi.org/10.1007/s11196-023-09990-1.

Modan, Naaz. "Supreme Court Says Schools Can Separate Athletics Based on 'Biological Sex,'" K-12 Dive, June 30, 2026,

Morris, Andrea. "Children's Show 'Odd Squad' Becomes Latest PBS Kids Show to Feature Same-Sex Marriage." CBN, July 17, 2022. https://cbn.com/news/us/childrens-show-odd-squad-becomes-latest-pbs-kids-show-feature-same-sex-marriage.

"National Society Daughters of the American Revolution." 2024. Daughters of the American Revolution. October 24, 2024.<https://www.dar.org/national-society/visitor-information>.

NBC News. "U.S. Naval Academy Hosts First Same-Sex Wedding for Maryland Couple." NBC News, May 10, 2014. https://www.nbcnews.com/news/us-news/u-s-naval-academy-hosts-first-same-sex-wedding-maryland-n102276.

Necessary, Terra. "7 Queer Superheroes That Were Straightwashed for the Screen." *PRIDE*, 28 Apr. 2020,

Nikolas, Akash . "The Pro-Gay Message Hidden In Every Disney Film." The Atlantic. The Atlantic, April 23, 2014. https://www.theatlantic.com/entertainment/archive/2014/04/its-not-just-frozen-disney-has-always-been-subtly-pro-gay/361060/.

Orwell, George. *1984*. 1949. Reprint, Boston: Houghton Mifflin Harcourt, 2013.

Oxford Languages mid 19th century: Psychiatrists from Greek psukhē 'soul, mind' + iatreia 'healing' (from iatros 'healer')

Petracca, Enrico, and Shaun Gallagher. Review of *Trust and reliance in the cognitive institutions of cryptocurrency*. *Mind & Society* 24, no. 24 (April 15, 2024). https://doi.org/10.1007/s11299-024-00302-z.

Powell, Josie. "16 Kids Shows with LGBTQIA+ Characters and Storylines." Care.com Resources, June 9, 2023.

Prairie Public. "Military Chaplains Raise Gay Marriage Concerns." Prairie Public NewsRoom, May 13, 2012. https://news.prairiepublic.org/2012-05-13/military-chaplains-raise-gay-marriage-concerns.

Ramsden, Edmund and Jon Adams, "Escaping the Laboratory: The Rodent Experiment of John B. Calhoun and Their Cultural Influence," *Journal of Social History* 42, no. 3 (2026): 761–97,

Raspberry, William. "Defining Deviancy Down." *The Washington Post*, 28 Dec. 1992.

Review of *Daniel Patrick Moynihan | United States senator and sociologist | Britannica*. www.britannica.com, June 26, 2026. https://www.britannica.com/biography/Daniel-Patrick-Moynihan.

Review of *D.O.S.E. : The brain's happy chemicals, explained.* Khiron Clinics, January 11, 2020. https://khironclinics.com/blog/the-brains-happy-chemicals-explained/.

Review of *Defining Abnormality: The Four D's and Cultural Context • Psychology Town*. Psychology Town, July 29, 2024. https://psychology.town/fundamentals-of-mental-health/defining-abnormality-four-ds-cultural-context/.

Sanburn, Josh. Review of *Houston Pastors Find Themselves in City's Crosshairs*. TIME, October 17, 2014. https://time.com/3514166/houston-pastors-sermons-subpoenaed/.

Singer, Paul. "West Point Chapel Hosts First Same-Sex Marriage." *USA Today*, Gannett Satellite Information Network, 30 Nov. 2012,

Sloane, J.P. -Biography-IMDb (Internet Movie Data Base),

Spencer, Christian. *Changing America*, 25 Aug. 2021, www. https://thehill.com/changing-america/enrichment/arts-culture/569376-in-shocking-twist-on-iconic-character-superman/

Sprague, MA, Carolyn . Review of Religion and Sexuality | EBSCO. EBSCO Information Services, Inc. | www.ebsco.com, 2023.

Sullivan, J. (2015, July 28). Boy scouts of America lifts decades-old ban on gay troop leaders. Abcnews. https://www.abc.net.au/news/2015-07-28/boy-scouts-lift-ban-on-gay-scoutmasters/6653268

The Advocate, (a homosexual and lesbian news magazine) May 26, 1971

The Bald and The Beautiful at DAR Constitution Hall (10/17/2026) Tickets

"The Facade of Medical Consensus – Chloe Jones." *Harvard Journal of Law & Public Policy*, 3 June 2025, https://journals.law.harvard.edu/jlpp/the-facade-of-medical-consensus-chloe-jones/. Accessed 18 Aug. 2026.

Thompson/Bethesda, Larry. "SEARCH FOR A GAY GENE." *Time*. Time Inc., 12 June 1995. Web. 05 Aug. 2014.

"Trixie and Katya Playing at DAR Washington DC - Bing." 2026. Bing. 2026. https://www.bing.com/search?q=trixie%20and%20katya%20playing%20at%20dar%20washington%20dc&qs=n&form=QBRE&sp=-ghc=1&lq=0&pq=trixie%20and%20katya%20playing%20at%20dar%20washington%20dc&sc=12-45&sk=&cvid=C132DD424AB44F5E93479CDE947C40AF.

University of Utah. "Sexual vs. Asexual Reproduction." Utah.edu, 2016. https://learn.genetics.utah.edu/content/basics/reproduction/

U.S. Department of Education Opens Three New Investigations into Michigan School Districts for Alleged Title IX Violations. U.S. Department of Education, June 18, 2026.

Volokh, Eugene. "What Percentage of the U.S. Population Is Gay, Lesbian or Bisexual?" *The Washington Post*, 15 July 2014.

Weiss, Madeline C., Filipa L. Sousa, Natalia Mrnjavac, Sinje Neukirchen, Mayo Roettger, Shijulal Nelson-Sathi, and William F. Martin. "The Physiology and Habitat of the Last Universal Common Ancestor." *Nature Microbiology* 1,no.9 (July 25, 2016). <https://doi.org/10.1038/nmicrobiol.2016.116.>

Wong, Curtis M. "Marvel Comics To Unveil A Gay 'Captain America' In Time For Pride Month." *HuffPost*, HuffPost, 17 Mar. 2021,

Zafar Iqbal, Muhammad, Mazhar Rafee Jam, Muhammad Saleem, and Mushtaq Ahmad. "True Hermaphrodite: A Case Report." *APSP Journal of Case Reports* 2, no. 2 (July 30, 2011): 16. https://pmc.ncbi.nlm.nih.gov/articles/pmc3418019/.

ABOUT THE AUTHOR

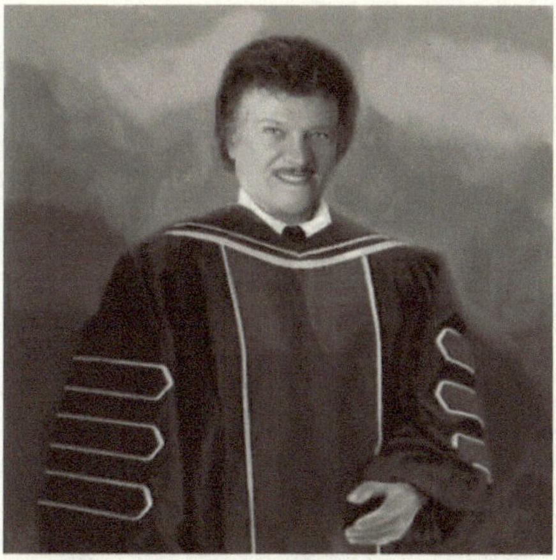

As a student of history, counseling, and theology, Dr. Sloane has researched not only the diversity of Christianity but also the various religions, sects, and cults to understand how they interact, challenge, and influence one another on all subjects. It was because of his quest for knowledge that Sloane pursued more than 30 years of higher education, graduating from The Master's University, where he earned a B.A., *Summa Cum Laude*, and an M.A. in Counseling. At Trinity Theological Seminary, he earned a Doctor of Ministry and a Ph.D. *With Distinction* in Religious Studies (world religions and cults).

Throughout the years, Dr. Sloane has appeared on many television and radio programs, including the 700 Club, Lester Sumrall Today, Richard Roberts Live, LeSea Broadcasting's Harvest, and Trinity Broadcasting Network's Praise the Lord, among others.

Publications in which Dr. Sloane appears include "Who's Who in the World" and "Who's Who in America." He is also featured in the "Dictionary of International Biography" and "2000 Outstanding Intellectuals of the 21st Century" (Cambridge, England).

www.ingramcontent.com/pod-product-compliance
Lightning Source LLC
LaVergne TN
LVHW090328210926
848480LV00004B/1332